THE WILDERNESS
FIRST AID HANDBOOK

THE WILDERNESS
FIRST AID HANDBOOK

Grant S. Lipman, MD, FACEP, FAWM
Clinical Assistant Professor of Surgery and Emergency Medicine,
Associate Director, Wilderness Medicine Fellowship
Stanford University School of Medicine

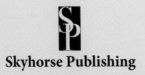

Skyhorse Publishing

Skyhorse Publishing books may be purchased in bulk at special discounts for sales promotion, corporate gifts, fund-raising, or educational purposes. Special editions can also be created to specifications. For details, contact the Special Sales Department, Skyhorse Publishing, 307 West 36th Street, 11th Floor, New York, NY 10018 or info@skyhorsepublishing.com.

Skyhorse® and Skyhorse Publishing® are registered trademarks of Skyhorse Publishing, Inc.®, a Delaware corporation.

Visit our website at www.skyhorsepublishing.com.

10 9 8 7 6 5 4 3 2 1

Library of Congress Cataloging-in-Publication Data is available on file.
ISBN: 978-1-62087-375-5

Printed in China

This book is dedicated to my father for introducing me
to wilderness medicine at an impressionable age,
my mother for her encouragement in all my endeavors,
and my wife, Ashlie, for her love, friendship, and
unwavering support for all my wilderness pursuits.

Acknowledgments

Thank you to all the wilderness first aid
instructors and staff at Stanford Outdoor
Education for their feedback,
Andy Fields for getting me involved and
for his constant enthusiasm, and Antja
Jean Thompson and Dr. Charlene Kiang
for all their assistance.

All illustrations by Willie Azali

CONTENTS

INTRODUCTION

People who work, live, travel, and recreate in the outdoors have specialized medical needs not adequately fulfilled by traditional first aid. Remote locations, arduous conditions, paucity of diagnostic and therapeutic equipment, and a need to make critical decisions often without outside communication have led to development of wilderness medicine as a specialty. These situations may be found in remote wilderness, the developing world, or in urban areas following natural disasters. This book is to be used as a guide to augment the skills and training learned in a typical wilderness first aid course. The intention is to assist the lay public, outdoor professionals, and instructors as well as members of wilderness first aid classes with useful and practical information that complements their training. Some elective skills are included, which the individual can decide to utilize depending on his or her comfort level and specific training.

This book is written for those who have basic first aid knowledge, not necessarily those with advanced degrees in medicine or pre-hospital care. The American Heart Association has limited components of their resuscitation curriculum, recognizing that some tasks may be difficult for laypersons to competently perform.

Similarly, this book acknowledges that certain knowledge and procedures are outside the scope of the average wilderness first aid provider's knowledge, and thus limits the use of technical terms or advanced techniques that may be unfamiliar to some readers or impractical based on the wilderness setting. This book provides easy-to-follow protocols and instructions to assist those encountering most wilderness emergencies.

While the contents of this book are meant to assist in managing a medical emergency in a remote environment, the information is generalizable to any setting where the reader is first on the scene. The protocols contained in this book are to be used as guidelines and by no means as a substitution for common sense or definitive medical care. A rescuer is liable for his or her own actions and should never undertake a medical procedure he or she is not comfortable with or which is not absolutely necessary, unless the rescuer believes the victim may lose his or her life or limb without intervention.

Most medicines discussed in this book can be purchased over the counter. Consult Appendix A for dosing specifics. Consult with a doctor concerning the potential side effects, complications, or contraindications of any medications you carry. Similarly, ensure that there are no known allergies to the medicines you use.

Travel in the wilderness is an inherently risky activity, as one often travels to remote locations for adventure, solitude, and serenity. Ultimately, the ethos of self-reliance found in the backcountry is epitomized by a wilderness medical emergency. These protocols assume knowledge and implementation of patient assessment systems that should not be ignored when acting on these protocols. Familiarize yourself with the information within these pages before venturing into the backcountry to minimize the chances that an accident will have to be an emergency.

⚠ This danger symbol next to the "red flags" of a patient's symptoms serves as an indicator of a dangerous disease process that may necessitate imminent evacuation to definitive medical care. If any of these red flags are observed, start early preparations for a potential evacuation. Consideration of the terrain, time of day, and weather are all potential issues in expediting a timely evacuation.

🚁 This helicopter symbol next to the "evacuate" assumes a medical emergency that requires a higher level of care via Emergency Medical Services (EMS). All evacuations assume the emergency is taking place in a setting where communication is likely not possible. The severity of the emergency, the potential for the patient to decompensate, the availability (or lack thereof) of outside communication, and the logistical and timely constraints of a rescue versus self-evacuation all need to be taken into consideration. **If patients are able to ambulate on their own without endangering themselves or others, self-evacuation may be a quicker and better option in the wilderness environment.** If a victim is unable to walk, or you expect that the ability to ambulate may shortly become compromised, you should likely send for a rescue. If the decision is made to send a messenger to initiate an EMS rescue, two people (buddy system) are better than one to ensure the safe delivery of both the message and messengers.

> **If the reader of this book is unsure of the necessity of an evacuation, err on the side of caution.**
> **"When in doubt, get out."**

ASSESSMENT SYSTEM

General Comments

Before you are able to administer first aid, an assessment must be made in an orderly process to ensure that both the rescuer and the victim are kept safe. First size up the scene, then undertake a primary followed by secondary assessment. If a problem is found, stop and fix it before moving on.

Scene Size Up:

- Ensure it is safe for the rescuer to approach the victim.
- Consider the number of victims
- **Mechanism of Injury (MOI)**. Consider how the victims may have injured themselves and their need for immediate spine immobilization (*see* **Trauma**).
- **Precautions.** If body substances are present, consider gloves prior to handling the victim.

Primary Assessment:

- Introduce and identify yourself as you approach the victim.
- Obtain verbal consent to treat them.
- Establish responsiveness.

- **Level of responsiveness (LOR): A-V-P-U**
  - Alert, Verbal, Pain, Unresponsive.

- **ABCDE**

- **A**irway
  - Open airway by the head tilt/chin lift.

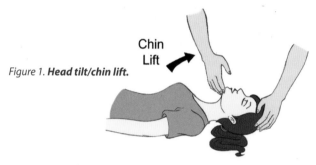

Figure 1. **Head tilt/chin lift.**

- Look in the mouth to clear any obstructions.
- Perform heimlich maneuver/abdominal thrusts if the person appears to be choking or there is an obstructing foreign body.

Figure 3. **Heimlich maneuver**

Figure 2. **Hands position for Heimlich maneuver**

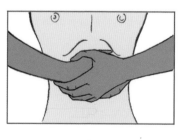

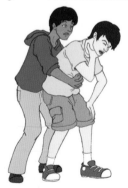

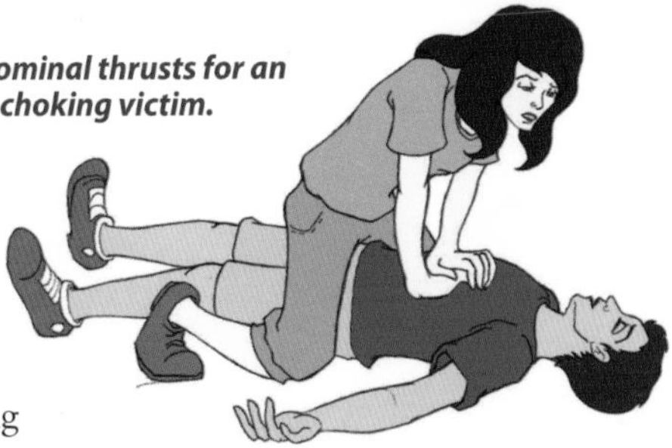

Figure 4. **Abdominal thrusts for an unconscious choking victim.**

- **B**reathing
    - Look and listen for breathing.
    - No breathing? (*see* **CPR**).
    - Assess if breathing is difficult or painful (*see* **Chest Pain, Chest Trauma,** and/or **Lung Problems**).

- **C**irculation
    - Feel for a pulse
    - No pulse? (*see* **CPR**).
    - If rapid pulse, check for site of bleeding (*see* **Wound Care**).

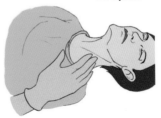

Figure 5. **Feeling for a pulse**

- **D**ecide/**D**isability
    - Consider the MOI and decide early if there is a necessity for spinal immobilization (*see* **Trauma**).

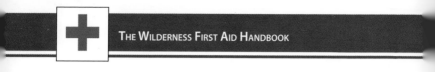

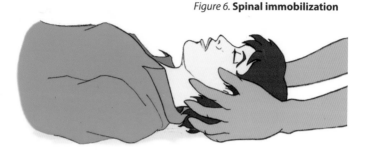

Figure 6. **Spinal immobilization**

- **E**xposure/**E**nvironment
  - Expose serious wounds for full evaluation and treatment. Consider environmental causes (heat, cold, lightning) as well as protecting the patient from further environmental stressors as treatment progresses (e.g., place on an insulating pad soon rather than later in the care).

Secondary Assessment

- Determine chief complaint
- History of the illness (how and when it happened)
- **SAMPLE** History
- **S**ymptoms
  - **A**llergies (to medications/latex)
  - **M**edications
  - **P**ertinent medical history

- **L**ast food or drink
- **E**vents relevant to the chief complaint.
- Check vital **S**igns: heart rate, respiratory rate
- Physical Exam: Ask where the victim hurts, look for wounds or injuries, feel gently the areas of concern, and check head to toe for injuries.

The SOAP Note:

Collect information and write it down as soon as possible. Document what you do and any changes to the patient. This is important for both patient care and to protect the first aid responder.

- **S**ubjective/**S**ummary
- **O**bjective/**O**bservations
- **A**ssessment of what you think is wrong and assess any changes to the patient.
- **P**lan what you are going to do and whether the patient needs an intervention or evacuation.

Figure 7. **Recovery position** (*see* **page 11**).

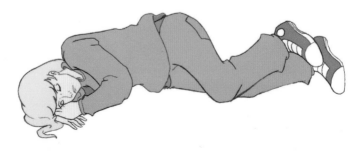

CARDIOPULMONARY RESUSCITATION (CPR)

General Comments

The standards for performing CPR are well established by the American Heart Association. CPR can be a life-sustaining intervention in the short-term, but the victim's survival rate after more than 20 minutes of CPR is very low. While CPR should be initiated when indicated, early alert of EMS for definitive care is of utmost importance. These CPR protocols are no substitute for taking a CPR certification class.

Contraindications to CPR in the Wilderness

Do not initiate CPR if there is:

- Patient responsiveness.
- Danger to rescuers, such that initiating CPR would put the rescuers at risk of harm.
- Obvious lethal injury (e.g., decapitation).
- A well-defined Do Not Resuscitate (DNR) status.

Discontinuation of CPR in the Wilderness

Once initiated, CPR should be continued until (any one of the following):

- Patient is responsive.
- The rescuers are exhausted or placed in danger.
- Patient care is turned over to EMS for definitive care.
- The patient does not respond to prolonged resuscitative efforts of greater than 20 minutes.

Figure 8. **CPR Schematic**

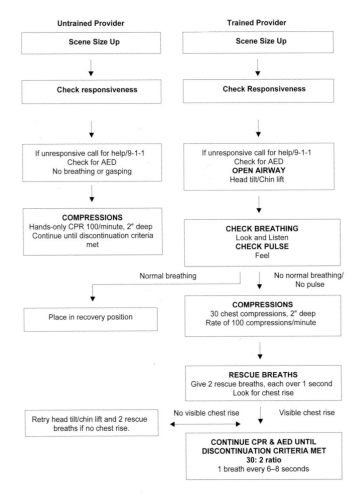

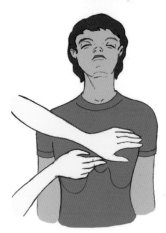

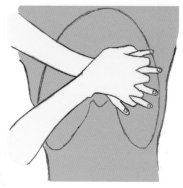

Figure 10. **Hand position for CPR**

Figure 9. **Hand position on the body for CPR**

Figure 11. **Body position for CPR**

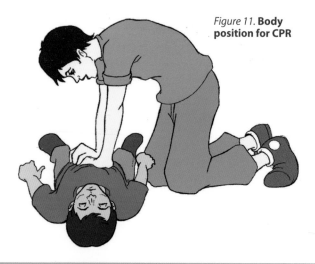

ABDOMINAL PAIN

General Comments

Abdominal pain is a potentially concerning, although not uncommon, complaint. Care must be taken in evaluating the patient for clues that may necessitate an evacuation for a problem that may require medical or surgical intervention. While this is a challenging problem in the backcountry, a thorough patient interview will be of great assistance in differentiating the diagnoses. Pay attention for red flags. Have a low index of suspicion to evacuate if pain persists for more than 12 hours. Evacuate any penetrating abdominal trauma.

Symptoms: Constipation (no stool for several days)

- Hard stools, bloating, distention.
- Crampy, intermittent, generalized pain.
- Pain may be greater in the left lower quadrant of the abdomen.
- Patient may be doubled-over in distress.
- **Red flags:** Presence of vomiting or fever with constipation, history of small bowel obstruction, or history of abdominal surgery.

Treatment:

- Maintain hydration with clear fluids.

- If dehydrated, rehydrate with electrolyte-containing fluids.
- Give caffeinated drinks (coffee, tea, hot chocolate) to stimulate the bowels.
- Give fiber or sips of mineral oil (if available).
- Give laxative (if available).
- Offer adequate bathroom time.

Symptoms: Nausea and vomiting and/or diarrhea.

- Crampy or sharp intermittent pain.
- Possibly associated with fever and/or fatigue.
- Diarrhea may be loose, watery, or with mucus.
- **Red Flags:** Diarrhea with blood or fever; vomiting with blood.

Treatment:

- Control the nausea with sips of herbal tea and Pepcid as needed.
- Rehydrate with electrolyte-containing solution. Start slowly (sips every 5 minutes), then when tolerating liquids, rehydrate until urine is clear.
- Ibuprofen or Tylenol as needed for pain.
- If mild diarrhea (4–6 stools/day), treat with Pepto-Bismol as needed.
- If frequent diarrhea (> 6 stools/day but no fever or blood in stool), treat with Imodium.

Symptoms: Lower abdominal pain in a female

- May be a dull or sharp pain, constant or intermittent, and may be one-sided.
- May include vaginal bleeding
- **Red Flags:** History of missed or irregular menstrual period, atypical from regular menstrual pain, one-sided pain.

Treatment:

- Ibuprofen or Tylenol as needed for pain.
- Pregnancy test.

Symptoms: Epigastric pain or "sour stomach"

- Pain at the top of the abdomen, may be burning, radiating up into chest or neck.
- Eating food or lying flat may worsen pain.
- **Red Flags:** Black tarry stools, bloody stools, fever, history of peptic ulcer disease, or history of heart disease.

Treatment:

- Pepcid and/or Pepto-Bismol as needed.
- Hydrate
- Cold water

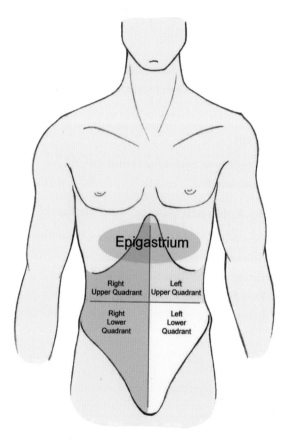

Figure 12. **Abdomen schematic**

Symptoms: Trauma (Blunt or Penetrating)

- Mild pain
- Nausea
- Pain worsened by flexing abdominal wall muscles
- **Red Flags:** Any hole in the skin or protruding bowel, pain that is progressively becoming more severe, pain worsened with any movement or palpation, pain in the shoulders after abdominal injury, bloating or persistent vomiting, fever, or any dizziness, rapid breathing, rapid pulse, or altered level of responsiveness.

Treatment:

- Sips of cold water
- Ibuprofen or Tylenol as needed for pain.
- Protruding bowel covered with clean moist (sterile) gauze with several dry layers of gauze affixed on top.
- Leave penetrating object in place and stabilized (*see* **Wound Care**).
- Have a low threshold for immediate evacuation.

Evacuate: Any patient with abdominal pain who also has:

- Abdominal pain worsened with movement.
- Persistent localized pain for more than 12 hours.
- Intermittent diffuse pain lasting more than 24 hours.

- Black tarry stools.
- Fevers > 8 hours with abdominal pain.
- Blood in vomit, stool, or urine (other than flecks of blood).
- Positive pregnancy test with abdominal pain.
- Inability to tolerate fluids.
- Any of the following: sunken eyes, dry lining of the mouth, decreased urine output, dizziness, and/or generalized weakness.
- Any penetrating trauma.
- Blunt trauma with red flags.

ALLERGIC REACTION & ANAPHYLAXIS

General Comments

An allergic reaction can be set off by exposure to a noxious stimuli like a bug bite, contact with a plant, or a food allergy. Symptoms of an allergic reaction range from mild to severe, the most severe of which is a life-threatening emergency called anaphylaxis. Most anaphylaxis will occur within 1 hour of onset of symptoms. Allergic reactions can recur (rebound), so it is imperative to continue the entire course of treatment. The incidence of true anaphylaxis is rare. Any patient who is suspected of having or who is being treated for anaphylaxis should be immediately evacuated. Epinephrine is reserved for cases of severe allergic reaction and/or anaphylaxis—this is a potent prescription drug, which can be dangerous to both provider and recipient. Administrators need to be trained in the unique delivery of the drug.

Symptoms

- **Mild:** Rash (may be diffuse)—red or blotchy skin, raised welts, itching, burning; red or watery eyes.
- **Moderate:** Skin rash and swelling to face or over entire body, sense of throat scratchiness or fullness, abdominal pain.
- **Severe/Anaphylaxis:** Shortness of breath, wheezing when breathing, tongue/lip swelling, hoarse voice, inability to speak, difficulty swallowing, and/or altered level of responsiveness.

• **Red Flags:** Any symptom of moderate or severe allergic reaction or anaphylaxis.

Treatment:

- Remove the offending allergen from the patient or the patient from the perceived offending trigger or environment.
- If a localized reaction, apply corticosteroid cream.
- **Mild and Moderate:** Benadryl (25 mg every 6 hours) and Pepcid (20 mg 2 times per day) for 3 days.
- **Severe/Anaphylaxis:** Hold EpiPen by grasping the shaft, and punch the tip into the outer thigh, releasing the hidden needle and delivery of medication. May repeat in 5–15 minutes if initial dose is ineffective or symptoms recur. Add all **Mild and Moderate** allergic reaction medicines.

Evacuate: Any patient who has received epinephrine. Any allergic reaction that does not improve with optimum treatment. Continue medications during evacuation.

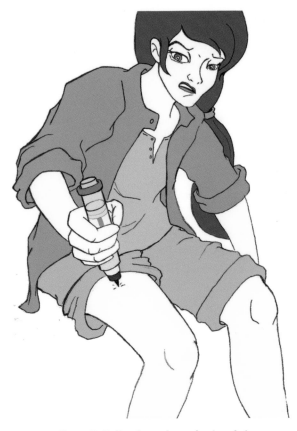

Figure 13. **Delivering a dose of epinephrine.**

ALTITUDE ILLNESS

General Comments

Acute mountain sickness (AMS) is the constellation of symptoms that results from the body's inability to adjust to the relatively low ambient oxygen concentration of high altitude. The compensatory response of the body upon ascending to high altitude is called acclimatization. Acclimatization is best accomplished by a gradual graded ascent with rest days. The body's **normal** response to high altitude includes increased urination; fast heart rate; fast breathing rate; swelling of fingers, hands, and feet; and intermittent rapid breathing while sleeping with brief breath-holding spells.

Altitude illness usually affects people traveling above 8,500ft—it is a spectrum of disease ranging from mild to severe AMS, high altitude pulmonary edema (HAPE), or high altitude cerebral edema (HACE). Mild to moderate AMS in the continental United States is most common. Remember that altitude illness may progress to fatal HACE or HAPE, so early symptom recognition and evacuation to lower altitudes may avoid a later rescue for a victim unable to walk or respond.

Guidelines for safety at high altitude:
- Ascend gradually to allow time for your body to naturally compensate to the physiologic stress of a low oxygen environment.

- When traveling above 10,000 feet, do not increase sleeping altitude by more than 1,650 feet (500 meters) elevation each night.
- For every 3,300 feet (1,000 meters) gain in sleeping elevation, take a rest day.
- If you feel sick at high altitude, assume it is altitude illness until proven otherwise.
- If you feel sick (mild symptoms) at high altitude, do not ascend to a new sleeping altitude until you feel better.
- If you feel sick (mild symptoms) and are unable to feel normal (acclimatize) after 24–36 hours, descend to the last elevation where you felt well.
- If you feel sick (moderate to severe symptoms) at high altitude, descend to the last elevation where you felt well.
- Altitude illness is often more severe the morning after ascent. This should be taken into account when considering evacuation decisions.

Symptoms

- **Mild AMS:** Headache, nausea, fatigue, insomnia, lack of appetite, dizziness—similar to a "hangover."
- **Moderate/Severe AMS:** More severe or pronounced symptoms of mild AMS.
- **HAPE:** Severe shortness of breath and/or rapid heart rate at rest or with mild exertion.
  - Dry cough, worse when lying flat (early in disease).

- - Wet cough, weakness, difficulty catching breath (later in disease).
  - Often begins on the second day after ascent to high altitude.
- **HACE:** Altered level of responsiveness, inappropriate behavior, seizures, lethargy.
  - Gait (walking) imbalance, loss of coordination.
  - Severe headache.

- **Red Flags:** "Ice pick" or "throbbing" headache on ascent, vomiting, any altered level of responsiveness, persistent elevated heart rate or breathing rate at rest.

Treatment:

- **Mild AMS:** Maintain adequate hydration and nutrition.
  - Ibuprofen for headache.
  - Do not ascend while feeling unwell.
  - Do not begin ascending until symptoms have completely resolved.
  - If symptoms do not improve in 24–36 hours, descend to last elevation where you felt well.
- **Moderate/Severe AMS:** Same as for mild AMS.
  - Immediate descent (at least 1,000 feet or until patient feels better).
  - If possible, do not wait until morning for descent.
- **HAPE/HACE:** Immediate descent, (at least 1,000 feet or until patient feels better).

- If possible and safe to descend, do not wait until morning.

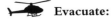 **Evacuate:**

- Any person who has HACE or HAPE.
- Never allow a sick person to descend alone.

BLISTERS

General Comments

Blisters are the most commonly reported injuries in the wilderness. While preventable and easily treatable, blisters can mean the difference between an enjoyable trip and incredible discomfort. Preparation begins with properly fitting footwear. Size the boots in the evening (when the foot is most swollen), and break them in before a trip to accustom both boots and feet to ensure comfort. Cotton socks should be avoided; a synthetic sock or a combination of thin synthetic inner sock and thicker cushioning outer sock has been shown to minimize blister occurrence.

Blisters start with **hot spots**—this sensation of heat is a warning sign that needs to be recognized and immediately treated to avoid progression to a painful blister. Treating a blister as soon as possible improves outcome and reduces potential complications. The pain of a blister arises from pressure on the incompressible blister fluid between skin layers. **Small blisters that do not cause discomfort should be left intact.** Otherwise, blister fluid should be drained to minimize discomfort and to keep the protective roof of the blister intact. The drainage and treatment of blisters is done in a way to minimize the possibility of infection. Blood-filled blisters represent a deeper injury and **should not** be drained. Likewise, blisters underneath calluses **should not** be drained, as they are painful to access, may incite infection, and re-accumulate fluid quickly. Keeping feet clean and dry (avoiding prolonged wetness) will lead to a lower incidence of blisters.

Symptoms: Hot spot

- Warmth, rubbing, discomfort, pain, or a raised red area. No fluid accumulation.

Treatment:

- Strip of paper tape over hot spot; the length should overlap the healthy skin on either side by at least the width of the hot spot. Take care to ensure no "dog ears" or wrinkles that may worsen the friction.
- **Prevention:** Apply paper tape to commonly irritated areas—pre-tape before starting your activity to prevent hot spots.

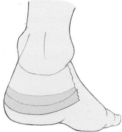

Symptoms: Blister

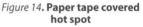
Figure 14. **Paper tape covered hot spot**

- Fluid-filled bubble of skin. Painful.
- ⚠ **Red Flags:** Blood-filled blister, redness/streaking around blister, blisters beneath a callus.

Treatment:

- Prepare both the blister skin and safety pin with an alcohol pad. The diameter of safety pin is larger than a sewing needle to allow continuous drainage, yet not too large as to risk de-roofing the blister.

- Puncture blister with pin at several points on the blister wall (towards the outside of the foot), rather than one large hole. This will allow natural foot pressure to continually squeeze out fluid, yet not make too large a hole that will destroy the integrity of the blister's roof.
- Gently push fluid out with your fingers or gauze.
- Blot expressed fluid.
- Cover with paper tape (protects the blister roof when removed), overlapping blister by double its diameter on either side.
- Can cover with benzoin (for adhesion), then shaped adhesive tape (such as Elastikon) overlapping the paper tape (twice the diameter of the blister). Trim tape with rounded corners to minimize dog ears and rolling off.
- Re-accumulated fluid can be drained through intact bandage.

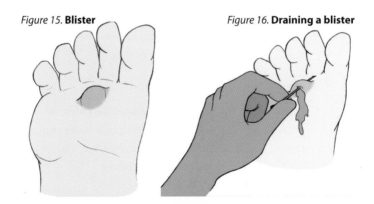

Figure 15. **Blister**

Figure 16. **Draining a blister**

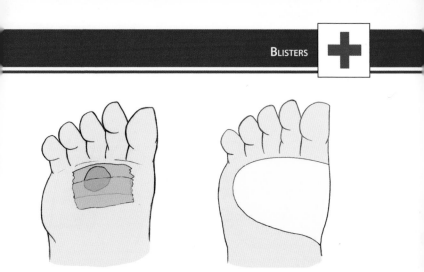

Figure 17. **Paper tape covering a drained blister**

Figure 18. **Elastikon tape covering a drained blister**

Symptoms: Open/Torn Blister

Treatment:

- Using small scissors, carefully un-roof the blister (painless), completely trimming off the dead skin.
- Place Spenko 2nd Skin to cover the raw area.
- Cover with paper tape.
- Can cover with benzoin (for adhesion), then shaped adhesive tape (Elastikon) overlapping the paper tape (twice the diameter of the blister).
- Trim tape with rounded corners to minimize dog ears and rolling off (as discussed with regular blisters).

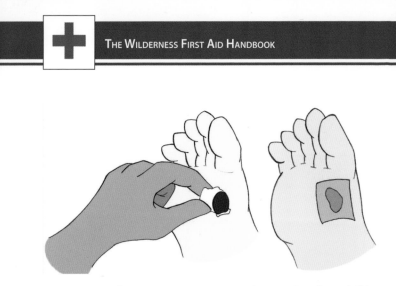

Figure 19. **Unroofing a torn blister**

Figure 20. **Spenko 2nd Skin covered open blister.**

Symptoms: Heel Blister

Treatment:

- Treat open or closed blister as described in the steps above.
- Shape the "heel cup" by taking a length of Elastikon (or other adhesive tape), cutting two midline incisions from either end, almost meeting in the middle, leaving a middle piece of tape intact. It will look like an *H* on its side.
- Trim all the corners.
- Apply benzoin for optimum adhesion.
- Apply the upper strip of the heal cup horizontally over the blister and intact skin above it.

- Wrap the lower two "wings" of the heel cup from under the heel up and perpendicular to the blister—with tension—anchoring the wrap.
- Trim off any corners or dog ears.

Figure 21. **Heel blister**

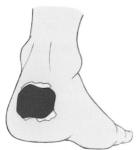

Figure 22. **Elastikon tape cut for a heel cup**

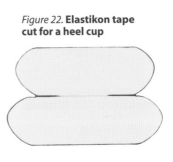

Figure 24. **Completed heel cup**

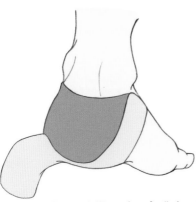

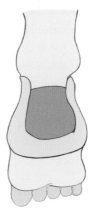

Figure 23. **Wrapping the "wings" of a heel cup**

Moleskin or Molefoam can be used on heel blisters to augment protection from a large blister. Cut a hole in the center slightly larger than the size of the blister, forming a donut shape, and place over the blister. Continue with all the steps previously listed.

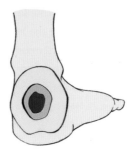

Figure 25. **Moleskin "donut"**

Symptoms: Toe Blisters

Treatment:

- Drain blister with prepared safety pin
- Apply one piece of paper tape along the top and bottom length of the toe.
- Use a second piece of paper tape to encircle the toe circumferentially (leaving tape end on top or bottom of toe to avoid irritating neighboring toes).
- Pinch closed.
- Trim sharp edges or wrinkles.

Figure 26. **Toe blister wrapped with paper tape.**

Avoid cloth tape or Elastikon on toes; abrasive tape will affect neighboring toes.

Toe pre-taping or hot spots can be wrapped the same way.

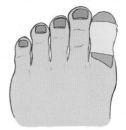

🚁 **Evacuate:** Few blister injuries require evacuation, unless it is too painful to walk or shows signs of an aggressive spreading infection (pain with redness, streaking, pus from wound, and/or fever).

Symptoms: Blister under toenail (subungal hematoma)

Swollen, painful toe nail, with fluctuance at nail base.

Treatment:

- Take an 18-gauge hypodermic needle and hold perpendicular to the nail area of greatest fluctuance.
- Rotate back and forth between thumb and first finger, applying downward pressure.
- Continue until blood oozes freely.
- If painful, stop.
- Put pressure on nail to squeeze out excess fluid.
- Recap needle, can reuse as these tend to recur.
- Wrap with paper tape like a toe blister.

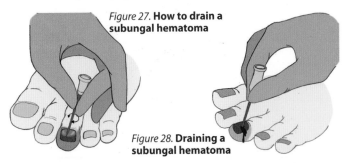

Figure 27. **How to drain a subungal hematoma**

Figure 28. **Draining a subungal hematoma**

BURNS

General Comments

Even small burns can be painful and debilitating. The most common burn in the backcountry is sunburn. Sunburn can be avoided by wearing hats, protective clothing, and use of high SPF sunblock with frequent reapplication. Like all wounds in the back-country, burns have the potential to become infected. Large burns should be considered for early evacuation for wound care and dehydration. Evaluate for any breathing difficulties that may represent a burn to the airway. Measure the size of a burn with your hand (palm of hand = approximately 1% of total body surface area), or per body surface area involved.

Figure 29. **Estimation of the burn size with the palm of hand**

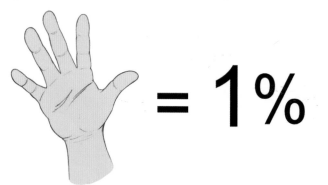

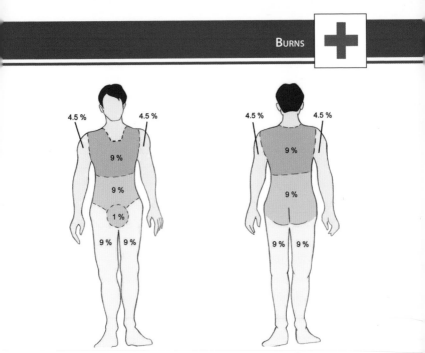

Figure 30. **Estimation of the burn size by body surface area.**

Symptoms

- **Superficial:** Reddened skin and pain (similar to a sunburn).
- **Partial Thickness:** Red skin and blistered; skin may be pale white/yellow, severe pain.
- **Full Thickness:** Flesh may be charred, no pain (nerve endings are burned).
 - **Red Flags:** Burns involving the face, lips, neck, hands, or genitals.

Treatment:

- Ensure the scene is safe.
- Extinguish burning clothes or material.
- Remove constricting clothes/jewelry.
- Immediately soak or flush the burn with cool water (ideally for 15–20 minutes).
- Wash burns with soap and drinkable water.
- Dress burn with antibiotic ointment and non stick gauze.
- Cover blisters with gauze dressing.
- Elevate involved extremity (to minimize swelling).
- Ibuprofen as needed for pain.
- Aggressive hydration.
- Monitor for infection. (Change bandage every day, observe for redness/streaking/pus from wound.)

Evacuate:

- Partial thickness burns involving more than 10% body surface area.
- Any full thickness burn.
- Any burn to the mouth, face, neck, genitals, and/or full circumference of any extremity: fingers, hands, or feet.
- Any burns > 10% of body surface area.
- Any burn that may have involved the airway (smoke inhalation), patient with cough, wheeze, singed nasal hair, or soot in nose or mouth.

CHEST PAIN

General Comments

Differentiating the causes of chest pain is difficult in the back-country with limited diagnostic tools at your disposal. Chest pain can be from an infection, a viral irritant, or a serious (and potentially fatal) problem in the lungs or heart. Ask if the patient has a history of heart disease or blood clots (or family history of this), or is currently taking medicine for high blood pressure. If so, assist him or her with taking prescribed medications. Younger people may complain of persistent rapid heart rate rather than pain. While it is better to avoid exerting a patient with concerning chest pain, it may be more timely and advantageous to have them ambulate to assist in the evacuation. If a patient has persistent chest pain—consider not moving the patient and bringing medical care to him or her.

Symptoms

- Chest pain, tightness, or pressure.
- Pain radiating to the left arm or jaw.
- Weakness, nausea, shortness of breath, and/or sweating with the pain.
- Lightheaded or dizzy.
- ⚠ **Red Flags:** Chest pressure that is worsened by activity, reduced by resting, and/or associated with sweating. Sharp, sudden onset chest pain with difficulty breathing.

Treatment:

- Reduce activity and anxiety. Place patient in a position of comfort.
- If patient has nitroglycerin, have him or her take as directed.
- Give Aspirin 325 mg (once per 24 hours).
- If symptoms occur at high altitude (>10,000 feet), reduce altitude by at least 1,000 feet.
- Younger patients with rapid heart rate should "hum" for 30–60 seconds.

Evacuate:

- Any patient with chest pain worsened by exertion or persistent chest pain (>20 minutes).
- Patient with persistent rapid pulse (> 100 beats per minute) or with associated shortness of breath and/or chest pain.
- If pain or shortness of breath is worsened by exertion, it may be of benefit to bring EMS to the patient rather than have them walk out in distress.

CHEST TRAUMA

General Comments

With trauma to the chest wall, injured ribs can be painful, but the primary concerns are injury to the underlying lung and blood vessels. Lung injury may have a delayed presentation after trauma, so careful observation is important for 12–24 hours after initial injury. Lung collapse can occur spontaneously with a sudden complaint of difficulty breathing and/or sharp chest pain, worsened on deep breaths.

Symptoms

- Reproducible chest wall or back tenderness on touching.
- Pain on taking a deep breath.
- Sensation of being unable to take a deep breath.

- **Red Flags:** Severe shortness of breath, passing out, "rice crispy" sensation over injury site, bubbles or gushing air exiting from chest wound.

Treatment:

- Place the patient in a position of comfort or on the non-injured side.
- For reproducible rib pain, wrap painful ribs with a circumferential ACE bandage (like a girdle), effectively "buddy taping" the area.
- Ibuprofen or Tylenol as needed for pain.

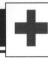
- Encourage patient to periodically take deep breaths (to inflate the lungs).
- If penetrating wound to chest with bubbles and/or air, affix gauze over wound, make an airtight seal by *taping on three sides* (leaving fourth side of bandage untaped to allow for air to exit).

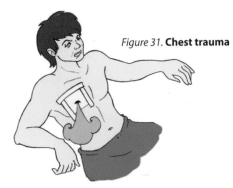

Figure 31. **Chest trauma**

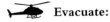 **Evacuate:**

- Any symptoms of difficulty breathing or shortness of breath after chest trauma.
- Coughing up blood after chest injury.
- Air bubbles/gush of air from chest wound.
- Cough producing sputum and/or fever.
- Persistent severe pain despite appropriate pain medicine and "buddy taping" chest wall.

COLD INJURY/FROSTBITE

General Comments

Cold exposure can cause both freezing and non-freezing injuries—depending on the depth of the skin layers involved. Frost-nip leads to numb, pale, soft skin whereas frostbite is the actual freezing of cells and a more severe cold injury. Cold injuries range from minor pain to extreme pain on rewarming and often permanent disability. Extremities are most prone to cold injury (ear lobes, nose, fingers, and toes). Factors contributing to cold injury include: hypothermia, prior frostbite, dehydration, constricting clothing/boots, wind, severity of cold environment, wetness, and concurrent alcohol or tobacco use. Rewarm/thaw the involved extremity as soon as possible to decrease eventual tissue damage, unless there is a chance of refreezing. Refreezing of the thawed extremity will worsen outcomes and the viability of affected tissue. It may be better to walk the patient out on frozen feet than to risk thawing and then refreezing the injury.

Symptoms

- Pale, white, waxy, hard skin, numbness (may feel like a "chunk of wood").
- Blanching of extremities (pinking of nail bed after pressure takes > 3 seconds).
- Blisters (clear).
- Mottled, dusky, "bluish" skin.
- After rewarming: Skin is swollen, red, painful.

- May develop clear blisters
- May develop blood-filled blisters (represents a deep tissue injury).
- **Red Flags:** Dusky mottled skin, blood-filled blisters.

Treatment:

- Primary treatment is the rapid rewarming of frozen extremity *only* if there is no risk of refreezing.
- Thaw with non-scalding water (104°F–106°F), should be hot-tub temperature.
- Keep affected extremity submerged for 20–30 minutes or until skin becomes soft and returns to normal color (may need to reheat water).
- Ibuprofen or Tylenol as needed for pain.
- Dress with gauze between fingers or toes and around extremity.
- Do not rewarm with radiant heat (fire).
- Do not massage or rub with snow.
- Blisters: drain clear blisters (*see* **Blisters**); *do not* drain blood-filled blisters.

Evacuate:

- Any patient with blood-filled blisters
- Dusky, blotchy, skin.
- If unable to use the injured extremity due to either pain or immobility.
- If unable to protect area from further cold or refreezing.
- Any patient whose pain cannot be managed in the field.
- Any signs of infection to affected area.

DENTAL PAIN

General Comments

Dental pain can be remarkably severe, but while potentially debilitating from discomfort, it is rarely due to a reason that will necessitate an evacuation.

Symptoms

- Extreme tooth sensitivity to hot/cold stimulus.
- Swelling to gum or cheek.
- Visually or palpably identifiable tooth irregularity.
- **Red Flags:** Severe swelling to gum or cheek.

Treatment:

- If a crown or filling is lost or the tooth breaks, cover the edge or "hole" with soft candle wax or sugarless gum, bite down to get a good approximation.
- Ibuprofen or Tylenol as needed for pain.
- Avoid very hot or cold liquid or food.
- If the tooth is knocked out of the socket, irrigate the tooth with drinkable water and attempt to replace it in the socket. Do not scrub the roots to clean. Make a "splint" of neighboring teeth using cooled soft candle wax. If tooth cannot be replaced, wrap in gauze and have patient carry the tooth between their cheek and gum.

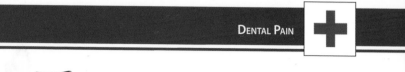

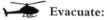 **Evacuate:**

- Any patient with a tooth knocked out of the socket.
- Any broken tooth with severe pain.
- Increasing swelling to cheek or gum.

DIABETIC EMERGENCIES

General Comments

Diabetes is a disease that is usually well-maintained and managed in the wilderness setting. Diabetic emergencies arise because there is a mismatch between the amount of sugar (glucose) in the blood and the body's ability to utilize that sugar (too much or too little insulin). **Diabetics in the wilderness setting should consider checking their blood sugar with frequency, as well as familiarizing the trip leader with personal testing apparatus and medicines.** The diabetic should plan ahead with the trip leader for optimum storage and administration of supplies (glucometer, spare batteries, syringes, ketone strips, and duplicate medications such as insulin, pills, glucose paste), and establish a sick day plan. Also plan to have routine meal times.

Insulin and cold: Avoid having insulin freeze. Keep next to skin in freezing temperatures, and if crystallized do not thaw or use.

Insulin and heat: Avoid prolonged direct sunlight and temperatures in excess of body temperature. Store wrapped within a sock next to a cool water bottle and/or in insulated case to retain coolness. Prolonged warmth may degrade efficacy of insulin, so test sugars more frequently.

Insulin is to be administered by the patient only.

If unsure whether a diabetic who has altered LOR is suffering from too little sugar or too much, it is better to assume a low sugar state and give sugar.

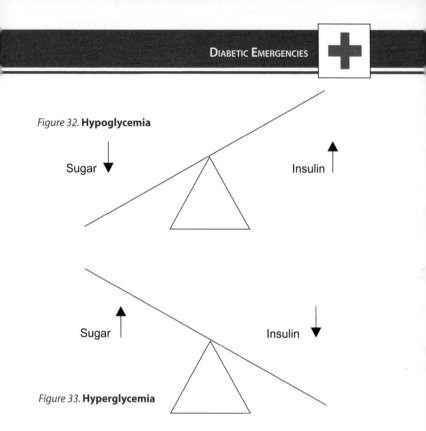

Figure 32. **Hypoglycemia**

Sugar ▼

Insulin ↑

Sugar ↑

Insulin ▼

Figure 33. **Hyperglycemia**

Symptoms

- **Low blood sugar:** rapid onset (minutes to hours)
    - Weak, sweating, confused, slurred speech, agitated, headache, seizure.
- **High blood sugar:** slow onset (days)
    - Fatigue, hunger, excessive thirst, excessive urination, abdominal pain, nausea, vomiting, and blurred vision.
    - Possible preceding infectious symptoms.

⚠ • **Red Flags:** Change in LOR, increasing thirst and/or urination.

Treatment:

- **Low blood sugar** (< 60 mg/dL)
  - Check blood sugar using the patient's glucometer.
  - If conscious, give sugar/sugar water/candy then complex carbohydrates.
  - If unconscious, rub sugar/sugar containing gel on inside of cheek or under the tongue.
  - Once patient regains consciousness, give food to maintain normal blood sugar levels (80–120 mg/dL).
- **High blood sugar** (> 300 mg/dL)
  - Check blood sugar using the patient's glucometer.
  - Aggressive hydration and evacuation.

Evacuate:

- Any patient with diabetes who has lost consciousness or has prolonged changes in LOR for more than 15 minutes.
- Persistent vomiting or diarrhea.
- Any person with diabetes who cannot (or will not) moderate his or her blood sugar levels.

EYES, EARS, AND NOSE

General Comments

Injuries to the eyes can range from the irritation of a speck of dust to a scratch on the outer covering of the eye, infection, or snow blindness. The most important thing with eyes is to note preceding trauma and/or history of contact lens use. Contact lenses predispose people to more severe infections. Nose bleeds or irritation to the nasal lining are often incited by trauma or dry air. Ear issues are often mild infections, usually caused by a virus, which may resolve on their own with pain control.

Symptoms: Eyes

- Foreign body sensation, pain, irritation, tearing, redness, sensitivity to light.
- Severe pain/light sensitivity 12 hours after extended exposure to bright/reflected sunlight (possible snow blindness).
- Specks or "floaters" in vision.
- **Red Flags:** Colored drainage from eyes, pain and redness in only one eye, loss of vision or new "floaters."

Treatment:

- If foreign body sensation, irrigate with drinkable water.
- If foreign body visualized, dab at it with moist, clean cloth.

- If painless appearance of blood in the white portion of eye, do nothing.
- If impaled object in eye, stabilize object with gauze padding and tape and patch both eyes.
- If possible "snow blindness" (sunburn to the eyeball), patch eyes/keep covered as needed for comfort. (If no sunglasses, consider using cloth/duct tape with small cut holes or slits to see through). Ibuprofen or Tylenol as needed for pain.

Symptoms: Ears

- Ear pain, tenderness to manipulation of external ear, foreign body sensation

Treatment:

- Ear should be flushed with warm water via an irrigation syringe.
- Ibuprofen or Tylenol as needed for pain.

Symptoms: Nose

- Bleeding from one or both nostrils

Treatment:

- Sit patient upright, then blow both nostrils hard to evacuate the clot. Pinch and hold the nose at the nostril crease. Hold constant pressure for 15 minutes. If unable to control bleeding, consider packing the nose with gauze (soak gauze in regular [non-herbal] tea to assist with constriction of the blood vessels).

- If mild nose bleed that stops on its own, consider applying antibiotic ointment inside nostril to lubricate the dry skin that may be irritated.

 Evacuate:

- Persistent eye pain, purulent discharge, severe redness to both eyes, or any vision changes.
- Eye redness/foreign body sensation in a contact lens wearer (which may signify a dangerous infection).
- Impaled object in the eye. Patient will have eyes patched and be unable to see or ambulate. Will need to bring EMS to the patient.
- Persistent nosebleed or nosebleed that requires packing.

FEMALE GENITAL PROBLEMS

General Comments

Most female gender medical concerns are manageable in a wilderness setting. Take care to create a comfortable environment that encourages participants to discuss these concerns with first aid providers. It is of primary importance to determine if the patient is pregnant (with lower abdominal pain and/or vaginal bleeding), as this will determine the need for an emergent evacuation to evaluate the pregnancy.

Symptoms: Vaginal bleeding

- Vaginal bleeding, painful menstrual cramps, bilateral or middle lower abdominal pain, pain 2 weeks prior to period.

Treatment:

- Pregnancy test.
- Ibuprofen or Tylenol as needed for pain.
- Hot water bottle to abdomen.

Symptoms: Urinary problems

- Burning on urination, increased frequency of urination, blood in urine.

• **Red flags:** Pain and tenderness to flank area and/or fever.

Treatment:

• Aggressive hydration

Symptoms: Vaginal burning, itching, discharge

Treatment:

• Wash vaginal area well, air dry well.
• Consider wearing cotton underwear, especially at night.

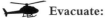 **Evacuate:**

• Any pregnant patient with lower abdominal pain.
• Any pregnant patient with vaginal bleeding.
• Symptoms of urinary problems that do not respond to therapy and/or persistent fever.
• Patient with pain or tenderness to flank area.

HEAD INJURY

General Comments

Patients suffering a head injury may initially appear well and oriented, only to later decompensate with an altered LOR. The first 24 hours after minor head injury are the most important to observe the patient for worsening symptoms, which may represent a more severe head injury and a neurosurgical emergency. Always consider the Mechanism of Injury (MOI) and possible spinal injury and necessary spinal immobilization precautions. Scalp lacerations tend to bleed a lot. Apply a bulky dressing of gauze compressed with a circumferential bandage or ACE wrap (*see* **Wound Care** section for closure of scalp lacerations).

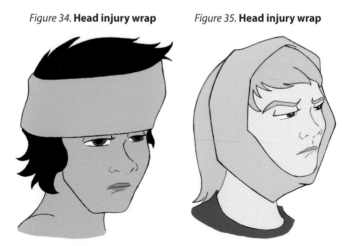

Figure 34. **Head injury wrap**   *Figure 35.* **Head injury wrap**

Symptoms: Minor head injury

- Headache, transient nausea and/or vomiting, "seeing stars," dizziness, mild LOR, or dazed. These symptoms should resolve quickly.

- **Red flags:** Loss of consciousness, rapid decompensation after initial injury (patient may appear drunk or have a change in normal behavior).

Treatment:

- Ensure that symptoms resolve quickly.
- Monitor for 24 hours to ensure no worsening of symptoms.
- Wake patient up overnight every 3 hours to ensure arousability.
- Ibuprofen or Tylenol as needed for pain.

Symptoms: Severe head injury

- Persistent symptoms of mild head injury that worsen in severity, blurred vision, lethargy, increasing disorientation, irritability, combativeness or otherwise altered LOR, persistent sleepiness, lack of coordination, seizures, persistent nausea, or vomiting.
- **Red Flags:** Black eyes or bruising behind ears, worsening symptoms of minor head injury.

Evacuate:

- Any patient with a loss of consciousness.
- Any patient with altered LOR.
- Any patient with symptoms of severe head injury.
- Any patient whose symptoms of minor head injury do not show improvement after 8 hours.

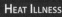

HEAT ILLNESS

General Comments

Heat-related illnesses might be due to overexertion, under- or overhydration, or medications that exacerbate the body's response to a hot environment. An accurate patient history may be more helpful than a thermometer. Overhydration with plain water while excessively sweating may lead to a dangerous depletion of the body's salt balance. Always rehydrate with electrolyte containing fluids and/or salty foods. Exertion in hot climates may expose one to heat exhaustion or heat stroke. A person is more susceptible to heat illness while on certain medications (some cardiac medicines, high blood pressure medicines, anti-anxiety/depressants, over-the-counter cold medicines, alcohol, stimulants) or in humid conditions. Cold water immersion is the best way to rapidly cool someone with heat illness—immerse up to level of nipples and be cautious to keep shoulders and head dry and secure in case of loss of consciousness.

Symptoms: Low salt level (hyponatremia)

- Weakness, nausea, dizziness, or muscle cramps.
- Altered LOR (without elevated temperature).
- Seizures.
- **Red flag:** Altered LOR, seizures.

Treatment:

- Rehydrate with dilute solution of sugar drink with salt or with an electrolyte solution.
- Provide gradual intake of salty foods.

Symptoms: Heat exhaustion

- Flushed, rapid pulse, sweating, dizzy, nausea, headache, chills, history of decreased water intake and/or decreased urine output.
- Crampy abdominal pain.
- **Red flags:** Dark yellow or bloody urine, decreased urine output, predisposing medications.

Treatment:

- Stop exertion and rest in shade.
- Rehydrate with electrolyte containing fluids.
- Gentle stretching for cramps.
- **Evaporative cooling:** Wet the victim's clothes/head and make a fan/draft to dissipate heat through evaporation.
- Cool with wet cloth.

Symptoms: Heat stroke

- Symptoms of heat exhaustion but with **altered LOR**
- Seizures
- Patient may be sweating or have dry skin, may be flushed or pale.

Treatment:

- Similar treatment for heat exhaustion with **aggressive** cooling: Cold water immersion is first choice (if available), otherwise, evaporative cooling.
- Cautious hydration of the patient with altered LOR, as they are at risk of seizures and subsequent vomiting and aspiration.

Evacuate:

- Heat stroke (or any altered LOR)—these should have EMS brought to them to minimize exertion and further heat generation.
- Persistent symptoms of heat exhaustion that do not improve.
- Red/brown urine.

HYPOTHERMIA

General Comments

Hypothermia occurs when the body's ability to produce and retain heat is overwhelmed by the cold effect. Wind and moisture lead to more rapid and severe heat loss. Hypothermia treatment has three main focuses: (1) minimize the effect of cold, (2) increase heat production, and (3) minimize heat loss.

The clinical presentation of hypothermia is more important than the patient's temperature, as it may be difficult to obtain an accurate temperature in the field. **Mild** hypothermia can effectively be managed, but any symptoms of **severe** hypothermia must be recognized early, as the wilderness setting offers limited reheating methods. The rescuer may be limited to minimizing cold effect and heat loss. Recognize that severe hypothermia will likely require evacuation and rewarming via EMS.

Symptoms: Mild hypothermia (90–95°F)

- Shivering (persistent).
- Loss of fine motor coordination (stumbling).
- Withdrawn or irritable, confusion, and/or poor judgment.

Treatment:

- Change the environment and find shelter.
- Replace wet clothing with dry clothing, add wind and waterproof layers.

- Add insulation under and around the patient.
- Cover head and neck.
- Hot/sweet liquids and food (calories).

Symptoms: Severe hypothermia (< 90°F)

- **Cessation of shivering** (at 86°F).
- Altered LOR, lethargic and may seem drunk.
- Combative or irrational.
- Slowed heart rate and respiratory rate.
- May appear in coma.

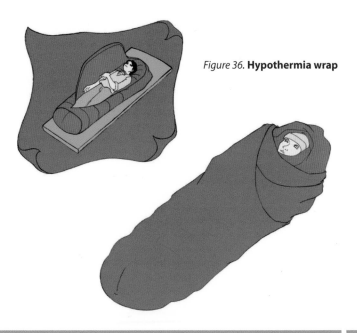

Figure 36. **Hypothermia wrap**

Treatment:

- **Evacuate**, as unlikely able to increase core temperature.
- Minimize heat loss and cold exposure. Wrap in sleeping bag with a warm hat.
- If altered LOR, be cautious giving fluids or food because of the risk of vomiting and aspiration.
- If in a coma, handle patient gently as heart is prone to fatal heart rhythms.
- Hypothermia wrap.

Evacuate:

- Mild hypothermia that you are not able to rewarm.
- Severe hypothermia.

INFECTIOUS DISEASE

General Comments

Viral "flu-like" illnesses are common and may be responsible for a spectrum of symptoms. While most of these symptoms resolve with time (a few days) and symptomatic care, the course of illness may be prolonged and require rest and an evacuation for complete recuperation. Ensure good hand hygiene before eating and after using the toilet (to minimize the viral spread and/or self-infecting). Do not ingest untreated water. Do not rinse fruit/vegetables in untreated water. Boil water before drinking.

Symptoms

- Nausea, vomiting, diarrhea, cough (productive or non-productive of sputum/mucus), fever, nasal congestion, sore throat, muscle aches, fatigue, headaches.

Treatment:

- General management for flu-like illness is treating the symptoms.
- Rest and rehydrate with electrolyte-containing solution. Start slowly (sips every 5 minutes), then when tolerating liquids, aggressively rehydrate with electrolyte-containing fluids.
- Control the nausea with sips of herbal tea, Pepcid and/ or Pepto-Bismol as needed.

- Ibuprofen or Tylenol as needed for headache, sore throat, muscle aches.
- If frequent diarrhea, Imodium.

Evacuate:

- Fever with headache, stiff neck, and sensitivity to light.
- Flu-like illness with persistent fever and/or difficulty breathing.
- Nausea/vomiting/diarrhea with inability to tolerate fluids for more than 12 hours despite medications.
- A sore throat with inability to swallow water and maintain adequate hydration (feels dizzy on standing and/or decreased urine output).

LIGHTNING

General Comments

Lightning strikes can affect many organ systems in the body, including: the heart (fatal rhythm), nervous system (bleeding in the brain, seizures, confusion, amnesia, temporary paralysis), the lungs (respiratory arrest), skin (burns), musculoskeletal system (dislocation or fractures), and eyes and ears (deafness or blindness). Initiate and perform CPR on any lightning victim who is not breathing and/or has no pulse, as their collapse may be due to a temporary breathing muscle paralysis (see CPR). The best defense against lightning is a good prevention plan specific to your geographic area.

Lightning Prevention

- If time between lightning and thunder is **30 seconds or less**, people are in danger of a strike and should seek appropriate cover.
- Wait at least 30 minutes after lightning/thunder before resuming outdoor activity.
- Seek shelter: big buildings, deep caves (3 times deeper than wide), metal vehicles.
- Avoid small shelters (e.g., tents), peaks, overhangs, and gullies that may increase risk.
- Avoid contact with metal objects and objects taller than you.
- Do not stand near isolated tall trees.

- Seek a low area near groups of small trees—**not** a clearing where a person may be the tallest object.
- If you are in the open, sit down in a lightning crouch.
- Sit on nonconductive padding (pack, pad, rope, life jacket).
- If in a **group**, spread out more than 20 feet, while maintaining visual contact (making sure that trip leaders are spread out as well).
- Get out of the water.
- Keep in mind: lightning can strike the same spot twice.

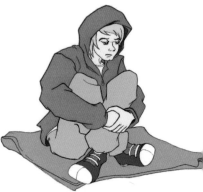

Treatment:

- Perform CPR if no pulse.

Figure 37. **Lightning crouch**

- If multiple victims require CPR, those with **burns to their heads** have lower rates of survival.
- Treat injuries as needed.
- Aggressive hydration.

Evacuate: Any patient struck by lightning, with a lightning burn or injury, or unconscious or change in LOR after nearby lightning.

LUNG PROBLEMS

General Comments

There can be many causes for shortness of breath, ranging from minor and non-life threatening (anxiety with hyperventilation) to diseases that may progress to a medical emergency (blood clot in the lungs, pneumonia). A thorough history may help you determine the underlying cause and likely indicate whether an evacuation is necessary.

Symptoms

- Rapid breathing rate.
- History of asthma or chronic lung disease.
- Wheezing.
- Numbness/tingling in the hands and feet.
- Worsening shortness of breath with activity.
- Chest pain associated with shortness of breath.
- Anxiety.
- Fever and cough with sputum.
- **Red flags:** Shortness of breath on exertion or with chest pain. Cough with shortness of breath, phlegm/sputum, and/or fever.

Treatment: Anxiety

- If the patient appears anxious with rapid rate of breathing, tingling in hands/feet (suspected anxiety attack), and no history of asthma, calm patient by being direct and reassuring.

- Give sack to breathe into.

Treatment: Wheezing

- If a history of asthma: assist patient with their own medicines (inhaler).
- **Severe:** Gasping with 3–5-word sentences, sweating, may appear fatigued or sleepy. Above medicines and EpiPen. May repeat in 5–20 minutes if initial dose is ineffective or recurrence of symptoms.

Treatment: Fever

- Cough with sputum, fever, and worsening shortness of breath, exacerbated by exertion—suspect pneumonia.

 Evacuate:

- Asthma attack not responding to the person's inhaler or requiring EpiPen.
- Asthma that does not resolve or worsens despite appropriate medication.
- Cough with fever and worsening shortness of breath.
- Shortness of breath associated with chest pain.
- Shortness of breath that worsens with exertion.

MALE GENITAL PROBLEMS

General Comments

Testicular pain after trauma is the most likely cause of male genital pain in the wilderness—the severity of pain dictates your ability to manage the patient. While infectious problems as well as surgical issues involving the blood vessels can be a challenge to differentiate, delay can result in loss of viability of the testicle, so the decision to evacuate for definitive care should be considered relatively early.

Symptoms

- Testicular pain.
- Often one sided.
⚠ - **Red flag:** Spontaneous severe testicular pain.

Treatment:

- Pain management with ibuprofen or Tylenol as needed.
- Elevation and support of the testicles.

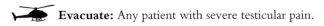 **Evacuate:** Any patient with severe testicular pain.

MUSCULOSKELETAL INJURIES

General Comments

The severity of the musculoskeletal injury in the wilderness setting is often dictated by the ability to use that extremity. A twisted ankle that cannot bear weight will require a similar treatment and evacuation as a broken ankle. If the injury is a direct blow or fall, always consider a broken bone. If the injury is from a twisting motion, a sprain, strain, or dislocation is more common. Look at the uninjured extremity to compare deformity, angulation, and overall appearance.

The most common dislocations are the shoulder, finger, ankle, and patella (knee cap), and all dislocations may be associated with a broken bone. Consider reducing a dislocation if you have specific training in the technique and if the patient is amenable to an attempt. In general, both the difficulty of reduction and the amount of long-term complications increase with delay in reduction attempts. Always check CSM—**circulation** (pinking of nail bed after pressure should take < 3 sec), **sensation** (dull versus sharp differentiation), and **movement**—and note if this changes after reduction attempt. All dislocation/reduction attempts should be done with calm and reassuring voice, applying slow, gentle, and constant effort (traction). If pain or resistance, go slower, maintaining constant traction and calming voice.

Symptoms: Broken bone

- Angulation or movement where no joint exists (a "false joint").

- Point tenderness on the bone.
- Inability to bear weight.
- Hear or feel grinding of bones together.
- Swelling or discoloration at the point of pain.
- **Red Flags:** Loss of CSM, angulation or tenderness to bony point.

Treatment:

- Remove jewelry.
- Pad bony points with soft material.
- If weight bearing/usable, suspect a sprain/strain, and apply compressive ACE wrap.
- If not weight bearing or patient is unable to use extremity, suspect broken bone, and apply sling or rigid splint (SAM splint).

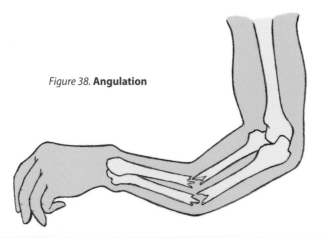

Figure 38. **Angulation**

- Sling/Splint: Immobilize joint above and below injured site in natural position.
  - **Wrist:** Splint in position like holding a beverage can.
  - **Ankle/Elbow:** Splint in 90° angle (rigid splint/sling/sleeping pad).
  - Secure firmly but not tightly.
- Ibuprofen or Tylenol as needed for pain.
- Check CSM before and after splint application.
- If open bone, irrigate copiously with drinkable water, and cover with antibiotic ointment soaked gauze.

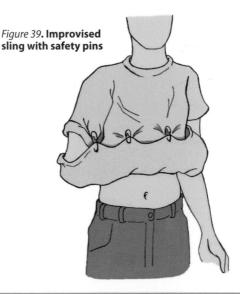

Figure 39. **Improvised sling with safety pins**

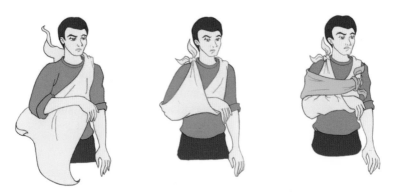

Figure 40. **Sling from fabric or triangular gauze**

Figure 41. **Appearance of dislocated shoulder**

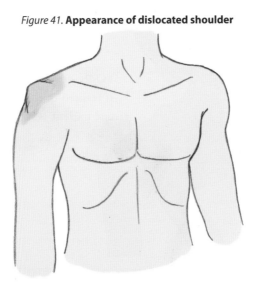

Symptoms: Shoulder dislocation

- Loss of natural curve of shoulder (shoulder appears squared)
- Holding affected arm up and away from body
- Unable to touch unaffected (opposite) shoulder with the fingers of the injured arm.

Figure 42. **Body position of a dislocated right shoulder**

*Only attempt reductions if trained in the procedure *and* patient is amenable.*

Treatment:

- Remove jewelry.
- Assess CSM.
- Reduce dislocation.
- If successful reduction, you will hear a "pop" and resolution of victim's pain.
- Recheck CSM and sling arm.

Knee-wrap reduction technique

- Sit the injured person down with bent knees.
- Clasp both the patient's hands around knees and have him or her lean back, slowly, until shoulder spontaneously reduces.

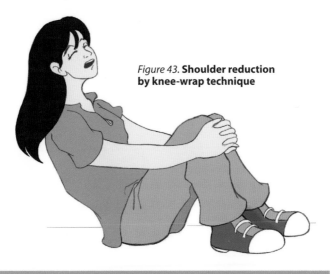

Figure 43. **Shoulder reduction by knee-wrap technique**

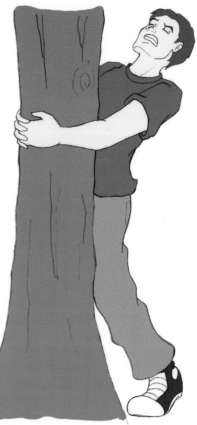

Tree-hug reduction technique

- Have the injured person wrap his or her arms around a slender tree (hugging it).
- Clasp both the patient's hands around trunk and have him or her lean back, **slowly**, until shoulder spontaneously reduces.

Figure 44. **Shoulder reduction by tree-hug technique**

Spaso reduction technique:

- Have patient lie on their back and, with calm and gentle voice and movements, grasp the injured arm by the wrist, holding straight up (perpendicular to the body).
- Apply gentle vertical traction while holding the arm straight.
- Keep patient relaxed as doing this, so the shoulder blade stays flat and in contact with the ground.
- Apply gentle external rotation (rotate toward the thumb side of the hand).
- After a few minutes of traction, reduction should occur.

Figure 45. **Shoulder reduction by Spaso technique.**

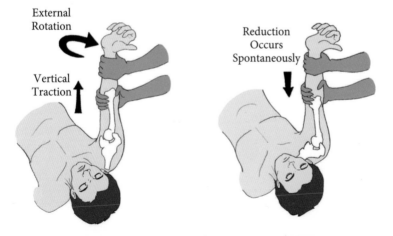

External Rotation Technique:

- Have patient lie on his or her back, and with calm and gentle voice and movements, have them bend their affected elbow at 90°.
- Holding affected arm above and at the elbow.
- Slowly bring the arm out and away from body.
- Rotate arm outward like opening a book (so back of hand and forearm is facing the ground).
- Bring arm up (like overhand throwing a ball), reduction should occur.
- Be patient; this process may take 5–10 minutes. If resistance is met or pain increases, stop movement, but don't let go.

Figure 46. **Shoulder reduction by external rotation technique.**

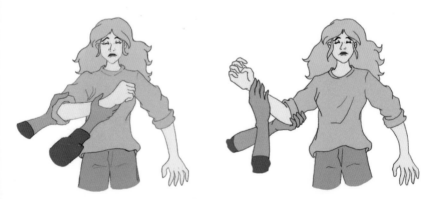

Symptoms: Kneecap dislocation

- Knee feels unstable/leg collapsed.
- Kneecap is repositioned to the outer aspect of the leg.

Treatment:

- Sit patient up, flexed at hip, making a 90° angle with the leg and torso.
- Straighten leg while pushing kneecap towards the midline (with continuous rapid motion).
- Hyperextend leg (bend the knee opposite of natural joint movement). Kneecap should pop back in.
- Post-reduction, patient can bear weight and walk out.
- Immobilize knee with sleeping pad/rigid splint and fashion "suspenders" to keep splint from slipping down.

Figure 47. **Kneecap reduction**

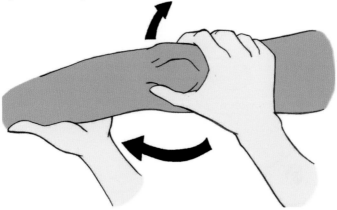

Symptoms: Fingers/Toes

- Fingers angulated at a joint.
- Unable to bend finger joint.

Treatment:

- Slow steady movement.
- Do not jerk.
- Pull with inline stabilization (pull the direction the finger/toe is pointing in).
- Pull until you hear a "pop" and joint appears to have normal orientation.
- Buddy-tape finger/toe (with adjacent finger or toe).

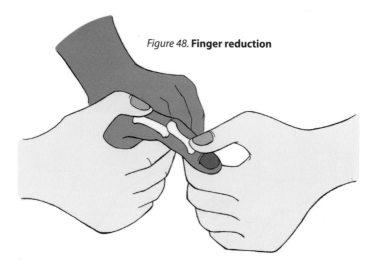

Figure 48. **Finger reduction**

Figure 49. **Finger buddy-taping.**

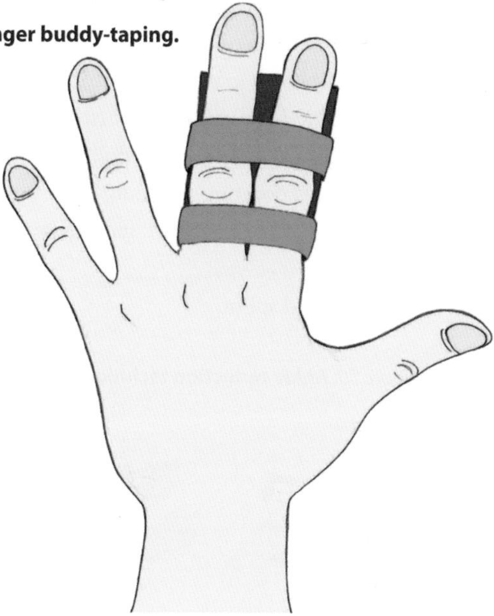

Symptoms: Ankle dislocation

- Angulation (often pointing out from midline).
- Bony protrusion/tenting of skin.
- Pain and inability to bear weight.

Treatment:

- Have patient lie down with affected leg bent at the knee.

- Have one person sit with back to patient holding/ stabilizing lower leg/calf (counter-traction).
- Have second person grasp mid-foot just below the ball of the foot (one hand) and at heel (second hand).
- Applying constant strong force, pull away from body in direction foot is pointing (traction).
- Once a release of tension is felt, guide foot back to midline.
- Check CSM and splint.

Figure 50. **Ankle reduction technique**

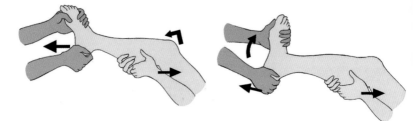

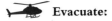 **Evacuate:**

- Any patient with an unreduced dislocation.
- Any patient with altered CSM before or after reduction.
- Any **unusable** musculoskeletal injury—whether a suspected sprain, strain, broken bone, or dislocation— either due to pain or joint instability.

NERVOUS SYSTEM EMERGENCIES

General Comments

Primary injury to the brain can present as a focal neurological deficit (weakness or numbness in extremities on one side), which may be transient or constant, and can present as bilateral lower extremity weakness (and progress up the body), as unconsciousness, or as a seizure. Patients with known seizure disorder (epilepsy) should be seizure-free for at least 6 months, carry own medicine, and cleared by own medical doctor before embarking into the wilderness. Seizures can occur as a primary disorder (e.g., epilepsy) or secondary to an environmental injury or other illness (e.g., low blood sugar, low salt level, heat stroke). If the patient does not have a known diagnosis of epilepsy, look for potentially reversible causes.

Symptoms: Neurological deficit

- Decrease in muscle strength on one side (arm and/or leg).
- Unsteady gait.
- Dizziness.
- One-sided facial droop.
- Headache leading to unconsciousness.
- Bilateral leg weakness/numbness progressing up the body.

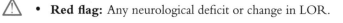
 • **Red flag:** Any neurological deficit or change in LOR.

Treatment:

- Place the patient in a position of comfort unless unconscious, then position patient in the recovery position.
- Thorough physical exam to document neurological deficits and any changes.

Symptoms: Seizure

- Patient feels encroaching seizure (aura).
- Blank staring gaze for few seconds.
- Localized extremity involuntary movement without loss of consciousness.
- Generalized shaking of entire body with unconsciousness.
- Incontinence of bowel/bladder.
- Altered LOR post-seizure.
- **Red flag:** Any seizure in a person without known epilepsy (first time seizure). Multiple seizures or prolonged duration than usual.

Treatment:

- Protect patient (move patient away from environmental hazards).
- Pad under head if generalized seizure
- If patient appears to be choking or turns blue, use head tilt/jaw thrust maneuver to open airway. Never put your finger or another object in a seizing person's mouth.
- Once recovered, position patient in recovery position.
- Perform complete physical exam to check for injuries.

Evacuate:

- Any patient with a focal neurological deficit.
- All seizures.
- Patient with epilepsy, who has multiple seizures without regaining consciousness, or a prolonged seizure (> 15 minutes).
- Any epileptic on trip who has had a simple seizure and is now going to potentially hazardous terrain (e.g., narrow cliff hiking, kayaking, etc.).
- Any patient with an altered LOR of unknown origin.

SKIN IRRITATION

General Comments

Take care to educate yourself on identifying toxic plants, such as poison oak, poison ivy, stinging nettle, and poison sumac. Many skin irritations can be prevented though improved hygiene practices and appropriate clothing. The active ingredient that causes the reaction is oil that can be transferred to the skin. Inhaled smoke from burning plants can also cause a reaction.

Symptoms

- Itchy red rash, fluid-filled blisters. Blisters may be delayed for several days.

Treatment:

- Rapidly wash the affected area (or suspected exposed area) well with soap and water.
- Wash all clothes and equipment that may have been exposed.
- Once the rash appears, itching can be relieved with of Hydrocortisone cream. More severe itching can be treated with Benadryl.

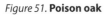

Figure 51. **Poison oak**

Figure 52. **Poison ivy**

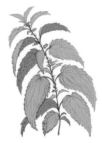

Figure 53. **Stinging nettle**

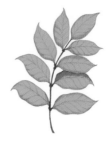

Figure 54. **Poison sumac**

🚁 Evacuate:

- Any reaction that involves the eyes, genitals, lips, mouth, or breathing.
- Skin irritation that is too uncomfortable to continue trip.
- Any signs of infection to skin (e.g., spreading redness, warmth, and/or pus).

SUBMERSION INJURY

General Comments

Always consider a traumatic injury (and possible spinal injury) in submersion victims. Be aware that inhaled water may have a delayed response on the lungs, leading to decompensation of breathing and a respiratory emergency hours after the initial event.

Symptoms

- Rapid breathing rate, shortness of breath, cough, wheezing, altered LOR, unconsciousness.
- **Red Flags:** Any breathing difficulties, persistent coughing (> 5 minutes).

Treatment:

- Ensure scene safety for the rescuer.
- Get patient onto dry land.
- Ensure spinal injury precautions.
- Initiate aggressive CPR (rescue breaths and/or chest compressions) if not breathing and/or no pulse.
- Be mindful of wet clothing, and initiate hypothermia preventive care early.
- Observe for any symptoms of breathing difficulty.

Evacuate:

- Any patient who lost consciousness during submersion.
- Any issues with breathing—shortness of breath, rapid breathing rate, "crackly" breathing sounds, blue discoloration around mouth—and/or altered LOR.

TOXINS, BITES, & STINGS

General Comments

The effects of an irritating toxin can range from a mild local reaction to critical systemic involvement. The inciting agent may be difficult to identify. Regardless, the goals of treatment are the same: minimize exposure, dilute (if possible), and maximize excretion of the toxin. Give symptomatic support, as specific antidotes are unlikely to be available in the wilderness environment. Fatalities due to bites, stings, or other envenomations are rare and may be due to anaphylaxis (*see* **Allergic Reaction**). While most bites and stings do not lead to more than a local reaction (or none at all), symptoms can worsen and progress, so evacuate *all* snake bites or scorpion stings.

Symptoms: Ingested toxin

- Mild nausea, vomiting, diarrhea, headache, collapse, seizures.

Treatment:

- Remove patient from offending toxin (e.g., tent with stove possibly causing carbon monoxide toxicity).
- Treat nausea and vomiting with sips of herbal tea and Pepcid.
- If absorbed toxin, wash off area with soap and water.
- If able, contact the American Association of Poison Control Centers (1-800-222-1222).

🚁 **Evacuate:** If the patient is unable to tolerate fluids, has persistent weakness, or collapses.

Symptoms: Snake bite

- Oozing at site, significant pain from bite, swelling, bruising, discoloration, possible shortness of breath, wheezing, numbness to mouth or tongue, muscle weakness, collapse.

- **Red flag:** Swelling or skin discoloration, any neurological symptoms.

Treatment:

- Remove constricting clothing and jewelry.
- Clean area and dress wound with antibiotic ointment.
- Mark site of initial bruising/swelling by circling with a pen.
- If difficulty breathing/wheeze, treat like anaphylaxis (*see* **Severe** under **Allergic Reaction**).
- Evacuate.

🚁 **Evacuate:** All snake bites, regardless of swelling or bruising, as symptoms may progress over 6-8 hours. Ambulate if able, otherwise send for EMS.

Symptoms: Stings or Bites (insects, bees, wasps, ants, ticks)

- Local pain, swelling, redness, weakness, nausea, vomiting, fever.
- Allergic reaction.

Treatment:

- Scrape off stinger.
- If tick is imbedded, grab the head with tweezers as near the skin as possible, and with constant gentle force pull up and away.
- Wash area well with soap and water.
- Cold compress to area.
- Benadryl for local inflammation/itching (*see* **Allergic Reaction**).
- If difficulty breathing/wheeze, treat like anaphylaxis **(**see **Severe** under **Allergic Reaction).**

Evacuate: Any sting with associated breathing difficulties or severe allergic reaction/anaphylaxis.

Symptoms: Spider bite

- Pin prick or painless bite, severe muscle cramps and pain in bitten extremity, may involve stomach or chest muscles, blistering or redness to site.

Treatment:

- Clean bite with soap and water.
- Ibuprofen or Tylenol as needed for pain.
- Cold compress to area.

Evacuate: If severe pain within 60 minutes of bite.

Symptoms: Scorpion sting

- Painful sting, burning pain to site, numbness to site, paralysis, muscle spasms, blurred vision, swallowing difficulty, breathing problems, slurred speech.

Treatment:

- Cool compress to site.
- Ibuprofen or Tylenol as needed for pain.

Evacuate: All scorpion stings. Symptoms may progress over 6–8 hours, evacuate early.

Symptoms: Jellyfish

- Skin irritation, severe burning, itching, nausea and vomiting, headache, muscle aches, dizziness, numbness, seizure, collapse, altered LOR.

Treatment:

- Rinse wound with seawater (avoid freshwater).
- Rinse with vinegar (avoid vinegar if suspected Man O' War).
- Make a paste of sand and water; scrape off extra stinging cells with edge of card/knife.
- Apply hot water *after* stinging cells have been scraped off.
- If allergic reaction or anaphylaxis, treat accordingly.

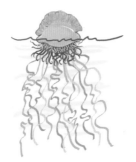

Figure 55. **Man O' War jellyfish**

Evacuate: Severe pain, any severe allergic reaction, or any breathing problems or neurologic problems.

TRAUMA

General Comments

The first premise in evaluating any trauma victim is to ensure the scene is safe for the rescuer; otherwise good intentioned assistance may lead to a second victim. Consider the mechanism of injury (MOI).

- Take *early* spinal precautions with patients prior to the **Focused Assessment of Cervical Spine (F.A.C.S.)**.
- Always ensure good breathing and a clear airway first.
- Have a second rescuer, if available, holding the cervical (neck) spine stability.
- Assume there is a spinal injury if a patient has altered LOR or unconscious.
- If necessary to roll a person (log roll) or move them to a safer environment, the movement should be coordinated by the rescuer at the head, ensuring the rolling/moving is done as a unit with as little side-to-side movement as possible.

Figure 56. **Spinal immobilization**

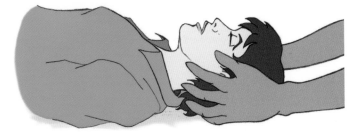

- Ask if any spine or back midline pain, weakness, or numbness to hands or feet prior to examination.
- Feel along the entire spine, looking for midline tenderness.
- If the person is conscious and reliable, the utilization of the **F.A.C.S.** can determine the presence or absence of an injury causing spinal cord compromise (which may lead to paralysis or death).
- If there is any suspicion for cervical spinal injury, err on the side of caution with full immobilization and then necessary evacuation.

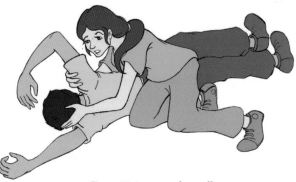

Figure 57. **1-person log roll**

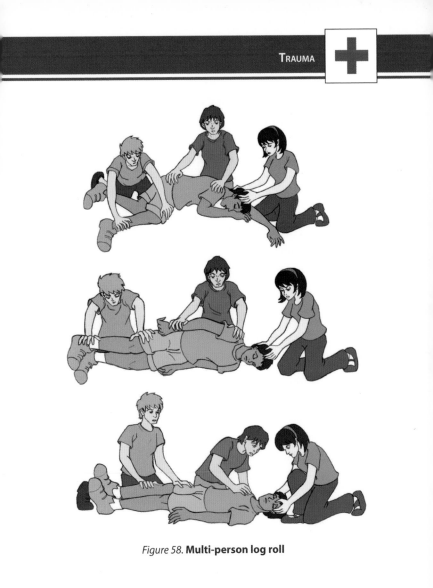

Figure 58. **Multi-person log roll**

Focused Assessment of Cervical Spine: F.A.C.S.
★Only perform if trained and comfortable with this
procedure.★

1) The patient is reliable: sober, alert, cooperative.

2) No strength deficits in hand grip, wiggle fingers and foot—push/pull.

3) No sensation deficits in upper or lower limbs (sharp versus dull differentiation).

4) No painful injury that may distract the patient from the presence of neck pain.

5) No tenderness to pushing on the upper (neck) middle spine.

★Check your F.A.C.S.★

If patient is alert, sober, has no point tenderness to midline neck vertebrae, has no sensation or motor deficits, has no distracting painful injuries, *and* can rotate head 45° to either shoulder and touch chin to chest without pain in the middle of the neck (side of neck pain is okay), you can "clear" the upper spine without need for a neck collar or further neck immobilization.

Treatment:

- Stabilize the spine by manually holding the head "in-line" with the rest of the body.

- Apply neck immobilization (e.g., molded SAM splint, backpack waist belt, etc.).

- Any log roll or movement done in small increments.

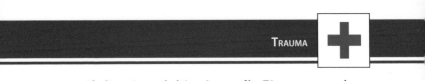

- If a litter is needed (*see* **Appendix B**) ensure to pad at bony points and under knees, with protection from the environment (e.g., cold, wet, sun), and removal of wet clothing.

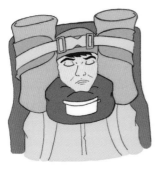

Figure 59. **C-spine immobilization**

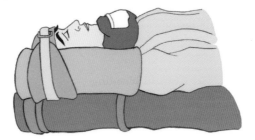

Evacuate: Any patient who has a possible spinal injury (cannot be cleared by **F.A.C.S.** or cannot walk due to pain).

WOUND CARE

General Comments

Wound management involves 3 steps: (1) control bleeding, (2) irrigation, and (3) wound closure. Try to use gloves when dealing with body fluids. Most wounds are simple and will stop with direct pressure and elevation—only very rarely are tourniquets indicated. Remember that any tourniquet may lead to eventual limb amputation, so use only as a last resort when life-threatening bleeding is occurring—when it's "*Life or Limb*." Any wound that occurs is at risk of getting infected. Copious irrigation is the first step to minimizing a poor outcome. Any water that is safe to drink is safe to flush a wound with. Finally, closing a wound may optimize aesthetic outcome but increases the risk of infection. Wounds that are not closed should be packed with gauze and allowed to drain and heal on their own.

Treatment:

1) Control bleeding

- Direct pressure (gauze bandage) for 10-15 minutes. Can use compressive ACE wrap.
- Elevate extremity above level of heart.
- Can apply a moist regular tea bag to wound to assist with bleeding control.
- If the patient has continued extremity bleeding despite the aforementioned methods, and there is concern that

they may bleed to death, consider a **tourniquet**. *"Life or Limb!"*

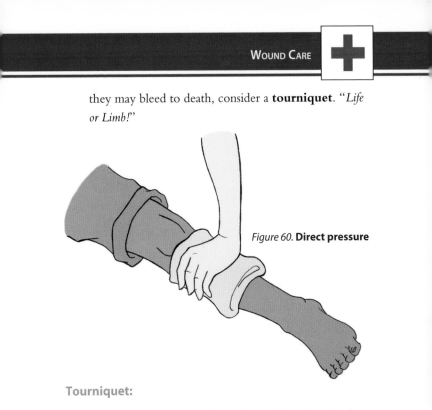

Figure 60. **Direct pressure**

Tourniquet:

1. Secure a band of cloth (at least 2" wide) 2" above extremity wound (between wound and the heart).

2. Tie half an overhand knot, put a small stick or rod on top of knot, and finish the half overhand knot over it.

3. Tighten tourniquet by turning stick until bleeding stops. Secure the stick (tape or another cloth knot).

4. Loosen the tourniquet in 20 minutes to check for bleeding. If bleeding continues, reapply tourniquet, noting time of application. If bleeding has stopped, leave tourniquet off.

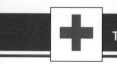

Remember: Applying a tourniquet may result in limb amputation

Figure 61. **Tourniquet**

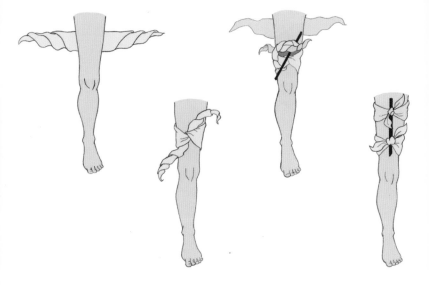

2) Irrigation

- Irrigate the wound with forceful pressure with an irrigation syringe, or poke a hole (diameter of 2 safety pins) in the corner of a plastic bag, squeezing water out onto wound, using at least 1 liter of drinkable water.
- Pull wound edges apart for thorough cleaning.
- Abrasions should be gently scrubbed with soap and water.

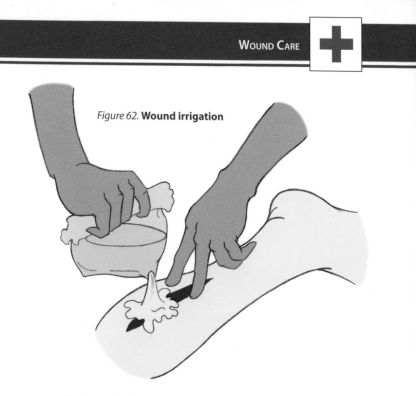

Figure 62. **Wound irrigation**

3) Wound closure

- Wounds with *edges that can be approximated may be closed*: Use wound closure strips or paper tape to tape the wound shut. Apply tape perpendicular to wound, opposing the edges. Apply another piece of tape and/or benzoin adhesive perpendicular to anchor the strips.
- Cover with antibiotic ointment and gauze dressing.
- Change dressing every 24 hours.
- **Do Not Close:** Puncture wounds, animal bites, or gaping or heavily contaminated wounds.

- **If needed, wounds may be left open** to minimize infection—such wounds should be covered with an antibiotic ointment–soaked gauze and then a wrap dressing.
- If wound is on joint of extremity, consider splinting wound.
- ⚠ **Red flag:** Signs of infection: pus, redness, streaking.

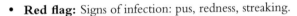

Figure 63. **Wound closure**

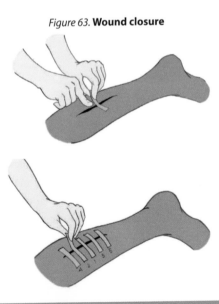

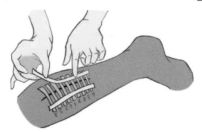

Scalp lacerations

- Take a strand of thread, fishing line, or thin string and lay it on top of (parallel to) the wound.
- Take strands of long hair on either side of the laceration and then cross them over, bringing the opposing wound edges together.
- Have another person tie a square knot with the thread as you hold the wound closed with hair.
- Repeat as many times as necessary down the length of the wound until the laceration is closed.

Figure 64. **Scalp laceration repair**

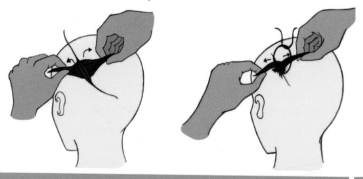

Impaled object

- Do not remove a large impaled object, as removal may lead to severe bleeding.
- Put a bulky dressing around the object to stabilize it.
- Secure the dressing well.
- Evacuate.

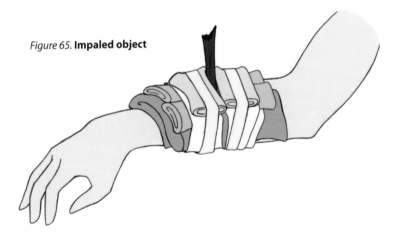

Figure 65. **Impaled object**

Fishhook removal

- Tie a string or shoelace around the bend of the hook.
- Push the shaft of the fishhook towards the barb/skin surface (this disengages the barb).
- Pull the string up and away at a 30° angle, yanking the hook from the skin with a snapping motion.

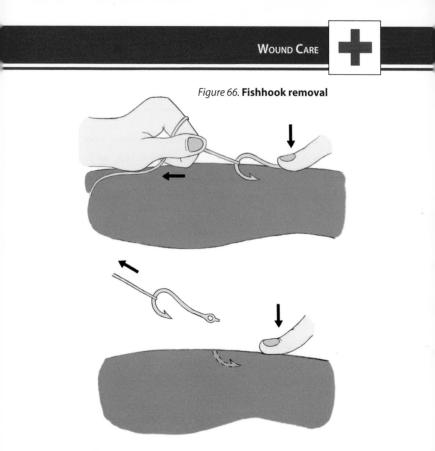

Figure 66. **Fishhook removal**

 Evacuate:

- Any amputation, tourniquet usage, or impaled object.
- Any wound that is heavily contaminated, involves a joint space, or which may involve underlying tendons or ligaments (loss of range of motion of hand, foot, finger, or toe).
- Any wound infection.

APPENDIX A. MEDICATION INFORMATION

Do not provide prescription medicine unless you are a physician, have been instructed by a physician, or feel that someone's life is in danger if you do not give the medicine. Always ask about allergies prior to dispensing any medicine.

In addition to having medication administration protocols, you should obtain informed consent for medication administration, even non-prescription medication. Inform the recipient of the indications, contraindications, and possible side effects of the medication, and obtain consent to administer. Before administering any medication read the protocols, confirm the dosage, read the label to confirm the medication, ask the patient about previous history with this medication and any known allergies, and ask the patient if they are currently on any medications and, if so, review the protocols for contraindications.

All dosing is indicated for adults. Listed medicines as generic names as well as commonly encountered brand names. Use of trade or brand names in this publication is for illustrative purposes only and does not imply endorsement by the author or the publisher.

Abbreviations:	PO	Oral
	IM	Intramuscular injection
	OTC	Over-the-counter
	Rx	Prescription

Medications

Pain Relief OTC

Acetaminophen	*(Tylenol)*
Ibuprofen	*(Advil, Motrin)*

Anti-Allergy OTC

Hydrocortisone cream	
Diphenhydramine	*(Benadryl)*
Famotidine	*(Pepcid)*

Anti-Allergy Rx

Albuterol	
Epinephrine	*(EpiPen)*

Antibiotic OTC

Polymyxin/bacitracin	*(Neosporin)*

Antidiarrheal OTC

Loperamide hydrochloride	*(Imodium)*
Bismuth subsalicylate	*(Pepto-Bismol)*

Anti-Nausea OTC

Famotidine	*(Pepcid)*
Bismuth subsalicylate	*(Pepto-Bismol)*

Pain Relief OTC

Acetaminophen (Tylenol)

Classification: Nonnarcotic pain relief, anti-fever.
Dose: 650–975 mg/4–6 hours PO (Maximum dose 4 g/24 hours)
Indications: For relief of pain due to headache, cold and flu discomfort, minor muscle and joint discomfort, and menstrual cramps. For reduction of fever. Especially useful for those allergic to aspirin or ibuprofen. Does not control inflammation.
Contraindications: Hypersensitivity, active alcoholism, liver disease, hepatitis. Acetaminophen is a common ingredient in over-the-counter pain, cold, and flu medicine. Be careful of accidental overdose in combination with other products.
Side Effects: Hypersensitivity rare

Ibuprofen (Advil, Motrin)

Classification: Nonnarcotic pain relief, anti-fever, anti-inflammatory.
Dose: 600–800 mg/6–8 hours PO
Indications: For symptomatic relief of pain associated with headache, colds, flu, frostbite, toothache, arthritis, burns, and menstrual cramps. May be used to reduce fever. For pain of inflammation and reduction of inflammation associated with muscle, joint, and over-use injuries.
Contraindications: Active stomach or intestinal ulcer, gastrointestinal bleeding disorder, history of hypersensitivity to aspirin or other non-steroidal anti-inflammatory drugs.
Side Effects: Nausea, abdominal pain, dizziness, rash

Anti-Allergy OTC

Hydrocortisone cream

Classification: Glucocorticoid (steroid)
Dose: Topical 1% cream, apply 2–4 times/day
Indications: For relief of pain and itching of jellyfish stings, poison ivy, oak, stinging nettles and sumac, insect bites, and other allergic skin reactions. May help dry oozing rash of allergic skin reactions.
Contraindications: Infections.
Side Effects: Itching, redness, irritation

Diphenhydramine (Benadryl)

Classification: Antihistamine (H1-blocker)
Dose: 25–50 mg/6 hours PO
Indications: For temporary relief of respiratory allergy symptoms and cold symptoms. Helps relieve the itching of allergic skin reactions. Useful in treatment of mild, moderate, and severe allergic and anaphylactic reactions. May be used as a mild sedative and for insomnia. May help alleviate seasickness.
Contraindications: Hypersensitivity, acute asthma attack, glaucoma, peptic ulcer.
Side Effects: Drowsiness, dizziness, weakness, dry mouth, thickening lung secretions, inability to urinate.

Famotidine (Pepcid)

Classification: Antihistamine (H2-blocker)
Dose: 20 mg/12 hours PO

Indications: For heartburn, acid stomach, and ulcer disease. Useful in treatment of "sour stomach," and moderate and severe allergic and anaphylactic reactions.

Contraindications: Hypersensitivity to famotidine or other H2-blockers

Side Effects: Constipation, diarrhea, dizziness, headache

Anti-Allergy Rx

Albuterol

Classification: Bronchodilator

Dose: 2 puffs of metered dose inhaler (MDI)/4 hours, or as needed.

Indications: Shortness of breath or breathing difficulty thought to be secondary to reactive airway disease (asthma) or anaphylaxis.

Contraindications: Fast heart rate secondary to underlying heart condition

Side Effects: Palpitations, fast heart rate, tremor

Epinephrine (EpiPen)

Classification: Bronchodilator, antiallergenic, cardiac stimulant

Dose: 0.3 ml 1:1000 IM, outside of thigh, repeat as necessary in 5–20 minutes.

Indications: For severe allergic reactions, including anaphylaxis and severe asthma attack.

Contraindications: No true contraindications with anaphylaxis, hypertension, cardiac disease, glaucoma, shock.

Side Effects: Increased heart rate, nervousness, dizziness, light-headedness, nausea, headache.

Antibiotic OTC

Polymyxin B sulfate (Bacitracin, Neosporin)

Classification: Antibiotic
Dose: Topical, apply 1–3 times/day
Indications: Contains ingredients for prevention of infection in minor wounds. Works as a lubricant, offers some relief from itching.
Contraindications: Hypersensitivity
Side Effects: Hypersensitivity reactions: burning, itching, inflammation, contact dermatitis.

Antidiarrheal OTC

Loperamide hydrochloride (Imodium)

Classification: Antidiarrheal
Dose: 4 mg PO (2 pills) initially followed by 2 mg PO after each loose stool (maximum of 16 mg or 8 pills per 24 hours).
Indications: For use in the control of diarrhea. Thought to limit peristalsis. Helpful in evacuating someone with severe diarrhea.
Contraindications: Hypersensitivity, bloody stool.
Side Effects: Dry mouth, dizziness, abdominal discomfort

Bismuth subsalicylate (Pepto-Bismol) chewable tablets

Classification: Antidiarrheal
Dose: 1–2 tabs PO every hour as needed (maximum of 16 tablets in 24 hours).

Indications: For use in the control of diarrhea.

Contraindications: Hypersensitivity to aspirin

Side Effects: Gray-black stool/tongue, nausea/vomiting, constipation, ringing in ears

Anti-Nausea OTC

Bismuth subsalicylate (Pepto-Bismol) chewable tablets

Classification: Antacid

Dose: 1–2 tabs PO every hour as needed (maximum of 16 tablets in 24 hours).

Indications: For use in the control of nausea.

Contraindications: Hypersensitivity to aspirin

Side Effects: Gray-black stool/tongue, nausea/vomiting, constipation, ringing in ears

Famotidine (Pepcid)

Classification: Antihistamine (H2-blocker)

Dose: 20 mg/12 hours PO

Indications: For heartburn, "sour stomach," and ulcer disease. Can be used in conjunction with phenergan for nausea. Useful in treatment of moderate allergic and anaphylactic reactions

Contraindications: Hypersensitivity to famotidine or other H2-blockers.

Side Effects: Constipation, diarrhea, dizziness, headache

APPENDIX B. EVACUATION INFORMATION

Daisy chain litter system.

Materials needed:
- Rope, at least 50 feet long
- Tarp or tent fly
- Sleeping bag or sleeping pad

Steps:

1: Lay out the daisy chain; loops are arms width (6'), with 15–20 loops.

2: Lay tarp and/or padding on the rope and package the patient.

3: Tie a loop knot with a bight (figure eight) at the foot end of the rope. Wrap the patient, cinching and looping each successive length towards the head, then tie off the rope.

Figure 67. **Daisy chain litter**

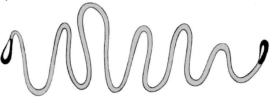

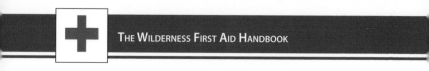

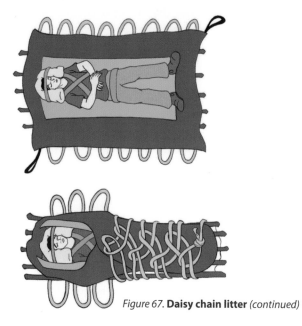

Figure 67. **Daisy chain litter** *(continued)*

Helicopter Rescue and Safety

Helicopter evacuation is generally considered when:

- The victim's chances of recovery are better with air than they are with ground evacuation.
- A ground evacuation would be arduous or unduly dangerous to either victim or the rescuers.
- The helicopter pilot and crew would be functioning within their safety protocols.

Information for helicopter team:

- Number of patients.
- Patient's weight and medical status
- Wind direction at landing zone
- Weather conditions at landing zone
- UTM or latitude/longitude coordinates and altitude
- Geographical description of landing zone

Do not fly conditions:

- Winds over 40 MPH (70 Km/hr)
- Night flight into mountainous areas
- Low visibility
- Poor or unknown landing conditions
- Slopes of more than 10°

Safety Rules:

- Never approach a helicopter until signaled to do so by the pilot or crew.
- Keep in line-of-site view of the pilot and crew.
- Stay clear of the landing zone and clear away debris prior to helicopter approach.
- Stand outside landing zone with back to the wind, facing the approach.
- Approach from downhill.
- Do not approach from uphill.
- Avoid the tail rotor.

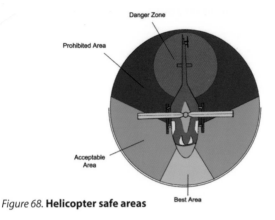

Figure 68. **Helicopter safe areas**

- Landing Zone Set-up:
    - Day: 100' x 100' (33 big paces)
    - Night: 150' x 150' (50 big paces)
    - Mark location/corners of landing zone with brightly colored objects/clothes that can show wind direction.

Figure 69. **Approaching a helicopter**

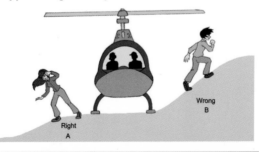

APPENDIX C. FIRST AID KIT

First Aid Kit:

- SAM splint
- Scissors
- Safety pins
- Duct tape
- Wound closure strips (¼" x 4")
- Benzoin (liquid adhesive) prep pads
- Alcohol prep pads
- Elasikon 4"
- Paper tape
- Spenco 2nd Skin (1" pads)
- Latex or nitrile gloves
- CPR microshield mask
- Q-tips
- 4" x 4" gauze dressing
- ACE wrap
- Sun block

Survival Essentials:

- Emergency space blanket
- Whistle
- Water bottle and water purification system
- Food
- Headlamp and batteries
- Map/compass/GPS

- Fire starter system
- Signal mirror
- Appropriate clothes/rain shell
- 7 mm nylon cord (accessory cord)—at least 30 feet